The Patient's Guide to

Periodontal Disease

By: Katrina M. Schroeder, D.M.D.

You have just had an exam at your dentist's office and been told that you have periodontal disease and that you need a special deep cleaning and all sorts of stuff that you have never had before. You are wondering why all this is important. Do I really need the deep cleaning? Why can't I just get a regular cleaning, the one my insurance pays for? Right now, this all seems like it is just a big expense that you had not planned for and are thinking that it is just a way for your dentist to make money.

I know this because I hear these same questions and comments from my patients every day. I understand. It is confusing. A lot of information has been suddenly thrown at you and you don't really know what any of it means. I have written this book for my own patients and made it available to everyone so that you can learn what this disease is and why your dentist is so adamant about treating it as well as what you can do about it.

First, periodontal disease is known in dentistry as the silent killer. Just as heart disease often shows very few symptoms until you suddenly have a heart attack, periodontal disease often has very few symptoms until it is in the more advanced stages. So you may not feel anything wrong, especially if yours has been caught early. There are, however, some things that you can look for.

Early in periodontal disease, you may notice that your gums are red and puffy around your teeth instead of smooth and pink. You may notice that your gums bleed when you brush and floss. You may have bad breath that does not seem to go away when you brush. For this last one, you may need to ask someone else that you trust, how your breath smells, because you usually cannot smell your own breath at all times. These are all symptoms of a problem with your gums.

In the later stages of periodontal disease, there are some other symptoms you can notice. Have your teeth moved in position? Do you have spaces between your teeth that you did not have before? Do your teeth wiggle? When teeth start to move like this, it means that they no longer have a strong base of gums and bone holding them in. Of course, there is always the end stage, have you ever had a tooth fall out whole, root and all?

Yes, periodontal disease is the silent killer of teeth. Periodontal disease, which is also called periodontitis, causes your bone and gums to detach from your teeth. This will eventually cause your teeth to fall out if you do not stop its progress. Most people would like to keep their teeth if they can. You have a disease that, if left alone, will cause you to lose your teeth while destroying the bone around them in the process.

But that is not everything that periodontal disease does. Periodontal disease is also linked to other killers: heart attacks, strokes, diabetes, even cancer. Yes, your dentist cares about your teeth and the health of your mouth. That is what they trained for after all. But these are why your dentist is up in arms to battle this disease. Your dentist wants you to be as healthy as you can be throughout your body and periodontal disease increases your risk of so many other detrimental diseases that it really needs to be addressed more, both in dentistry and medicine.

About this guide

I or my team review periodontal disease with my patients in the office every day. Here we have pre-made diagrams and models that we can show our patients. I will often draw out sketches of teeth for my patients as well. We tell my patients about their disease, they experience the diagnosis in their exam. We review the oral and systemic complications of this disease with them. And we give them a plan to treat their disease.

And we do it fast.

We throw a ton of information out to you, hoping that you will catch most of it.

Most people only catch a tenth of what we tell them. Well, we do give you a written treatment plan, so that is concrete and much easier to remember when you get home. The rest just swirls around in a big ball of confusion.

Some people ask us questions later as they come in for future appointments. Some people call and ask. Some people look things up on the internet, which has information all over the place, some of it old, some of it completely false, and some information that is dangerous and can damage your gums and your health. These patients often wind up even more confused than they started.

I have written this for you; to take that big jumble of information that was thrown at you and sort it out so you can understand what periodontal disease is, how to handle it, and why it is so important.

I have broken this book into sections for you to help you through your treatment. I start with what periodontal disease is and how it is diagnosed. Then take you through the first step of treatment and how to take care of your teeth at home. These are important things to get you started on your road back to health.

Then I will help you through the additional information that has been heaped upon you. I will review how your mouth connects to the rest of your body and how periodontal disease increases your risk for other diseases and complications including: heart disease, stroke, arteriosclerosis, and diabetes, low birthweight and pre-term babies, osteoporosis, Alzheimer's, and cancer. I will cover some of the advanced treatments, such as directly placed antibiotics, laser aided treatment, and surgical options. Lastly, I will cover peri-implantitis, which is the same disease around dental implants.

At the end of this guide, you will find a periodontal dictionary that gives you definitions of the technical terms used throughout the guide for you to use while reading and when discussing your care with your dentist.

So, let us continue on so you can learn about your periodontal disease and how you can control and improve your health.

What is periodontal disease?

Periodontal disease is a complex disease process that is a combination of a bacterial infection and a chronic inflammatory response. Yes, I know, that is a mouthful of an explanation that does not really get you any closer to understanding it.

I will start you where periodontal disease starts, at your gums where they meet your teeth. You were not born with periodontal disease. No one is. Your mouth is healthy, so that is where we will start, with a clean, new, healthy mouth.

The bacteria that cause periodontal disease, and the bacteria that cause cavities as well, do not stay in your mouth if they do not have teeth or something to stick to. They do not stick to your gums. You may have some get into your mouth from exposure to other people, but until you grew your first baby tooth, your saliva just washed them away.

This may seem like a long time to go back to, but it was the only way to start everyone with a clean slate.

Then your teeth grew in. And the contagious bacteria took hold. Yes, periodontal disease, and the bacteria that cause cavities, is contagious. You catch them from other people, usually your family. Just something for you to think about the next time you are around some young people that you are related to and fond of, how clean is your mouth and how many bacteria do you have in it to spread to these young people? How many bacteria do you have for them to catch?

Now, you are young and have just caught the bacteria that will, one day, cause your periodontal disease. The thing is; these bacteria do not cause periodontal disease immediately. This is just the initial infection. First these bacteria set up shop on your teeth. They group together and secrete a sticky goo to hold themselves onto your teeth. This goo forms plaque, that whitish goopy stuff you can easily scrape off with your fingernail, although a tooth brush is better and more hygienic than your nails.

This is still a healthy mouth that you have. Yes, you have bacteria in there stuck to your teeth that are potentially harmful, however, these bacteria, in low amounts and with the right mix of bacteria, also help you to keep fungus from taking up residence in your mouth. Going back to before your teeth came in, when you were a baby, have you heard of thrush? Thrush is a fungus called Candida albicans. Babies do not have strong immune system yet and they do not have good bacteria to help keep the fungus away. That is why babies are more prone to getting thrush.

This pre-disease state when your mouth was still healthy, and the bacteria levels just needed to be kept low, that is when you would have had preventative cleanings at your dentist's office. Preventative cleanings are meant to prevent periodontal disease and just keep your bacteria at low healthy levels. These are the cleanings that most insurance cover completely.

Most children and many adults are in this healthy state where we work to prevent periodontal disease. Periodontal disease is very rare in children, usually associated with some genetic abnormalities. Young adults, however, can have periodontal disease and have it be the same periodontal disease as usually found in older adults without needing a genetic susceptibility.

Now, I have been referring to these as just bacteria. Periodontal disease is caused by a group of bacteria, not just one. These bacteria include P. gingivalis, C. rectus, B. forsythus, and A. actinomycescomitans. That last one is a big baddie, because it is the primary culprit in childhood periodontal disease because these children are genetically unable to fight that one off. So you have a group of bacteria, working together, against you.

Actually, the bacteria are not specifically working against you. They are just living their happy little goo and acid producing lives. It is a problem when the bacteria build up to high enough levels that your body has to respond to it. Very low levels of them are ok. But when there are too many of them, then your body tries to fight them off.

The level of bacteria that it takes to trigger your body's fight response varies by person. That is why some people seem to have issues as young adults and some people seem to never have any issues. The level can also change within a person's lifetime. Medication changes, hormone changes, stress, life changes, aging, they can all lower your threshold for triggering the fight response.

So, what is this fight response that your body launches? It is inflammation. This is what causes the problems for you. Normally, your body launches an immune system attack, causing inflammation in an area of infection or injury. The problem with periodontal disease is that the bacteria are outside of your gums, stuck to the outside surface of your teeth. Your immune system gets right to the edge of your gums, almost to the surface, but it cannot get outside of your gums.

It gets stuck. And it gets angry. Your gums get red and swollen and irritated. This is inflammation brought by your immune system. This is gingivitis. Your gums are mad. They do not like the bacteria sitting right next to them because there is just too much of it. Your immune system has been called in and is biting at the bit to get at those bacteria and break them up and get rid of them and the sticky acid goo that they make, but it just can't get there.

Think of a castle, filled with knights ready to go, mounted up on their horses, all shining in their armor. Swords are drawn; pikes in hand. Now picture their enemy, a massive sea of people, not particularly combative, but there are a vast multitude of them, camped out there around the city and growing in numbers. They have been taking from the food supply of the country, skimming a little bit off each time a supply comes in. They were tolerable when it was just a few of them, what with being charitable to the downtrodden and all, but now they are a great host. And that great mass of people is making a lot of trash and a lot of waste. And they are throwing it against the walls of the castle. And they won't stop. They have been asked to stop, asked to leave, but they won't. And those knights are waiting in the castle, ready to go and make them leave, clean up their garbage that has filled the moat, kill if they have to. But the drawbridge is stuck closed. So all the knights can do is yell and get angry until their faces turn red.

That is what is going on with gingivitis. Red angry gums that are upset with the crud of biofilm being made by bacteria just next to them. Biofilm is the technical term for bacteria mixed with the sticky goo of plaque that they secrete to stay stuck to your teeth. Gingivitis is still reversible; you can make it go away. You just have to get rid of most of the bacteria and their sticky mess. Then, keep the bacteria away. This is easiest with the help of your dentist and hygienist for the first big cleanup, and then keep it clean so that the bacteria cannot build back up again. Sometimes, this cleanup can still be the preventative cleaning that insurances cover, sometimes this cleaning will need to be a bit more, based upon how much buildup of bacteria you have above and below your gums.

That is the part that makes periodontal disease difficult, the bacteria that make periodontal disease happen get into the space between your gums and teeth. Your gums form a little cuff around your teeth.

This natural pocket is supposed to be there. This pocket, called a sulcus in healthy areas, is shallow. It gives your gums right at the edge where they meet your teeth a little mobility to help keep them from being damaged by the foods you eat. Normally, this cuff is snug against the side of your teeth, but when your gums become inflamed, the gums swell, which pulls the gums away from the teeth and opens that pocket up so food and bacteria can get down in there. This is then even harder to clean, which leads to even more swelling. Yes, even when these shallow pockets are open and inflamed in gingivitis, a tooth brush and floss can still reach the bottom to clean it out, as long as it has not calcified.

Let us go back to the castle filled with knights surrounded by a crowd that is making a mess everywhere. You already know that those people, the knights enemy, has been piling up their garbage and waste in the castle moat and up the walls, well, after they have been doing that for a while, and the knights have not come out of the castle to clean things up, they start mixing concrete and pouring the concrete onto the trash piles before it sets and using the concrete trash mixture to build homes for themselves, making it even harder to remove them. Now, even if the people were removed, the sticky nasty concrete reinforced homes remain, making it easier for the people to hide and re-populate the area outside the castle.

This is what happens in your mouth. The bacteria make sticky goo from their waste that helps them bond to your teeth. They use a little bit of everything you eat to do this. When food is left in your mouth, it will turn into plaque in twelve to twenty-four hours. Plaque is the sticky bacteria filled biofilm goo. It is plaque when it is more bacteria than food. Plaque, just like food, is still removable with a tooth brush and floss.

After your food has been turned into plaque by the bacteria, it starts to be reinforced with calcium. Your saliva naturally contains calcium. It is there to re-mineralize your teeth after you eat acidic foods. It will also mineralize the plaque, turning it hard and tough. The bacteria love this, but your gums hate it. The calcification of plaque takes another twelve to twenty-four hours. Once your plaque has calcified and become calculus, you can no longer take it off with a tooth brush and floss.

Looking at the total time frames, for food to become plaque is twelve to twenty-four hours and for plaque to become calculus is another twelve to twenty-four hours. So, from food to calculus, that you cannot remove, is twenty-four to forty-eight hours. If you ever wondered why your dentist told you to brush at least twice a day and floss at least once, this is why, so you get everything cleaned off every day. If you miss a spot, for even as little as twenty-four hours, it can be covered in calculus that you can't remove.

Once calculus forms in one area, the conversion times become even faster. When an area already has a little spot of calculus, food becomes plaque faster and plaque becomes calculus faster.

All of this can be happening and you could still have just gingivitis, just inflammation that is still reversible. But then something changes. It could be that the bacteria build up even more, beyond what your gums can tolerate. It could be a new medication you take, or increased stress, or illness, or a hormone change lowers your body's tolerance level. That is what starts periodontal disease.

Back at the castle, the king, who is also trapped in the castle with his knights, has had enough. Something really ticked him off. Maybe he did not sleep well, or his shoe lace broke. It does not matter, the king is mad. The knights cannot get out of the drawbridge, so he orders them to go down into the dungeon and dig out the moat, make it deeper. If they can't kill off this messy, filthy hoard, they can try to separate themselves as much as they can. They can make the moat deeper so that there is somewhere for all of the sticky garbage to go so it does not overwhelm the walls. So the knights, being the dutiful knights they are, go down and dig the moat deeper. They still can't get out to remove the hordes of people outside the castle because of the cement reinforced garbage pile above them. Little bits of it fall down onto the knights as they dig the moat deeper. Occasionally, someone from the hoard that has been living in the cement reinforced garbage falls into the deepened moat too. That person then continues to just do what he was doing before, breeding and making a mess, while the moat is being dug ever deeper around him.

As the knights dig deeper and deeper, the castle now sits on a skinny pillar supporting its massive weight. Sometimes it is stabilized a bit by the concrete filled garbage at the top of the moat, but that it not very strong compared to the solid earth that once supported it. The castle on its skinny pillar begins to sway and rock in the wind, barely noticeable at first, but then more and more. The knights at the deep dark bottom of the moat that have been digging can't see it move because of all the garbage that has filled in above them. They just keep digging, following their orders to dig until the garbage is gone. Until one day when there is not enough support for the castle and it topples over.

Periodontal disease does exactly this to your teeth. When your body has an infection that it cannot get rid of, it tries to physically separate itself. The bacteria are stuck to the surface of your teeth, so your body pulls your gums away from where they attach to your teeth. And not just your gums, under your gums, your teeth are attached to your bone by a periodontal ligament. Your body pulls this back too, removing the surrounding bone with it while the swelling of your gums continues to get bigger, which makes it look like your gums have not moved at the early stages, even though the bone loss has already occurred. Your bone and gum attachment to your teeth continues to decrease and your pockets become deeper and deeper until your teeth fall out.

This happens around all of your teeth, but not at the same speed and at the same time. Some of this has to do with how well you clean the area. Front teeth are easier to clean than back teeth, but they also develop calculus faster. So this is why some teeth can be worse than others, even in the same mouth.

The inflammation of your gums does more than just cause your bone and gums to detach and erode away. It also causes complications throughout your body. Inflammation in one area of your body sends out chemical signals to the rest of your body, setting off chain reactions everywhere. This is how periodontal disease harms the rest of you.

How do you know when all of this is happening? How do you know your moat is getting deeper? Remember, swelling can keep the top edge of your gums is a fairly normal position until the depth has reached moderate to severe levels. Periodontal disease is diagnosed based off of several findings from a dental examination.

In a typical examination at my office, a series of x-rays (radiographs) are taken, different ones dependent upon your teeth, and a visual examination and periodontal charting are completed. In the visual examination, I start with a visual oral cancer screening, and then I look at your teeth.

As a side note, I do a visual oral cancer screening on all of my patients. Most dentists do, but some may not tell you that they are doing it. I usually tell children I am looking for anything strange going on rather than state that it is a cancer screening.

For most of my patients, I am reviewing their radiographs while my hygienist is completing their periodontal charting. Sometimes I will compete a patient's periodontal charting myself. I have been told that I am fairly gentle with this, but my hygienist is gentler than I am. Dental hygienists are licensed dental care professionals that have specialized in just the various non-surgical methods of cleaning teeth techniques as well as measuring and monitoring the health of your gums.

So, what is periodontal charting? It is measurements of where your gums and bone attach to your teeth, recording if you have bone loss below the furcation of your back teeth, if any teeth are mobile, and if your gums bleed or have any puss around your teeth. I know, you are wondering what a furcation is.

Your back teeth have more than one root. The

furcation is where the roots join together. If you think

of the roots of a tooth as legs, the furcation would be

the crotch. When your gum and bone attachment has

exposed the furcation, it is much more difficult to clean.

Periodontal charting uses a special instrument

called a perio-probe to measure how deep your

periodontal pockets are. There are a variety of styles of

these. Mine have markings every millimeter. Some

have markings at different intervals. Some even

connect to a computer to measure electronically. Your

dentist and hygienist will use the one that works best

for them.

The perio-probe is slipped into your periodontal

pocket and slid to the bottom of the pocket to measure

it. This takes very little pressure, but might need some

wiggling, dependent upon how much calculus and debris we have to get around. The perio-probes are completely blunt, but the calculus and debris in your periodontal pockets may be rough and scratchy, kind of like sand. If the measurements are uncomfortable for you, please let your dentist or hygienist know and topical anesthetic gel or even a local anesthetic shot can be used to numb the area so it is more comfortable. Most of my patients do not need to be numb or just choose the numbing gel to make it more comfortable. In my office, I prefer to say the measurements out loud to my assistant, who records them into your chart. That way you can hear where your deeper areas are as I go along through your teeth.

These measurements are the depth of your periodontal pockets. Generally, lower numbers are better. Measurements of one, two, and three millimeters are depths that you can keep clean with a tooth brush and floss. Most of the time, these are healthy or have gingivitis. Measurements of four are a warning. These areas your gums are swollen and some of these four millimeter areas have early attachment and bone loss. These are almost always areas with gingivitis. Measurements of five, six, or more almost always have attachment loss and periodontal disease.

I did write almost always because there are some medical conditions and medications that can cause your gums to grown so much that they cover over your teeth. If you have one of these, you probably know it already. In these cases, you could have deep areas without attachment loss, but would need to have the excessive gum tissue removed instead.

Once you have measurements of five or more, we know that you have bone and attachment loss, but how bad is it? Early periodontal disease is

measurements of five to six millimeters. Moderate is

six to seven millimeters. Severe periodontal disease is

greater than seven. You can have different severities in

different areas of your mouth, and sometimes on

different areas of one tooth. In any case, the greater

the severity in any area, the worse your prognosis for

the tooth, and the greater your risk of having

complications elsewhere in your body.

Your diagnosis is also based upon other findings

too. X-rays (radiographs) show some of your bone

levels, such as if your bone has receded to expose your

furcations, and if you have very dense older calculus.

The visual examination allows your dentist to see

inflammation, redness, and swelling of your gums as

well as areas of recession and exposed root surfaces.

All of these are combined to determine your diagnosis as well as your prognosis for your mouth. Which teeth are involved? How bad is it on any particular tooth? Is it that bad all around the tooth or just one part of the tooth? This is what I look for.

Your first step of treatment – Scaling and Root Planing

The first stage in fighting periodontal disease is scaling and root palning. This is one of several types of cleanings that can be completed in a regular general dental office.

A quick note on the other cleanings that are common. A prophylactic cleaning is one that is preventative; it keeps a healthy mouth healthy. It is also the cleaning that most dental insurances cover completely. A gingivitis scaling is a cleaning for people who have gingivitis, inflammation of the gum tissue without bone loss, spread throughout their mouth. These people do not have periodontal disease yet and the goal of this scaling is to help return them to a healthy mouth and eliminate the gingivitis. A full mouth debridement is for people who have so much plaque, calculus, and debris stuck to their teeth that their teeth cannot be seen to be accurately examined. In other words, this is for people who have so much stuff on their teeth that I cannot see their teeth. There are other types of cleanings as well that I will cover in advanced and adjunctive treatments.

Back to scaling and root planning. This type of deep cleaning goes into your deep, infected periodontal pockets and takes out the debris, plaque, and calculus. The goal is to get the level of bacteria down to levels similar to a healthy mouth so that the inflammation in your gums can subside. This cleaning also smooths the surface of your root so that it is easier for you to keep clean afterward, similar to polishing the tops of your teeth.

This process can be uncomfortable, and how uncomfortable it is depends upon how bad your periodontal disease is, how inflamed your gums are, as well as equipment and techniques used. It is up to you if you want topical (non-needle) numbing or if you want local anesthetic (shots) or if you prefer not to be numb at all. Most of my patients choose topical numbing so that it takes away some of the discomfort but they do not have to have shots.

Scaling is the part where the debris, plaque, and calculus are removed from your teeth. Root planning smooths the root surface so it is easier for you to keep clean, just as the tops of your teeth are polished in a regular cleaning or at your follow-up appointment. Both actions are done concurrently using specialized instruments to reach your deeply infected pockets.

There are two main types of instruments used to clean your teeth: hand instruments and ultrasonic instruments. Lasers are also sometimes used and will be covered under advanced and adjunctive treatments.

Hand instruments are entirely manual. They are thin instruments, shaped to fit against the roots of your teeth that slide into your infected pocket and pull out the bacteria. They have one side with a very sharp edge that shaves the bacteria off of your tooth root. Ultrasonic instruments use ultrasonic sound waves to break up the debris containing bacteria and a water stream to wash the debris away. While the hand instruments have been around for a very long time, the ultrasonic are a bit newer, they were invented in the 1950's, if you consider that to be new. Your dentist or hygienist will use one or the other or both, depending upon the needs of your teeth. Both are equivalent in more shallow areas, however, studies have shown that the ultrasonics are more effective in deeper areas.

Usually, directly placed antibiotics are recommended to be put into your infected periodontal pockets right after the scaling and root planning has been done. These are also in the advanced and adjunctive treatments were I will cover the different options. These directly placed antibiotics are put directly where the infection is. Even though the areas have been cleaned, they are still not sterile. Unfortunately, as soon as we clean an area out, bacteria from the rest of your mouth start to move back in. That is where the antibiotics come in. These do two things for you. First, they kill bacteria, with some of the antibiotics being effective for four weeks. Second, they fill the pocket so that food and other debris can't get in, an effect that can last for up to two weeks. This gives your gums a better opportunity for the inflammation to calm down and your gums to snug back close to your teeth.

A note about insurance, most dental insurances do not cover directly placed antibiotics, however, your medical prescription plan may. Medical insurances do not often work directly with your dentist; usually, your dentist fills out a prescription form, which you sign as well, and sends that to the antibiotic manufacturer. The manufacturer then contacts your medical insurance and handles the process from there. The process for this can take several days, usually because of a wait for your medical insurance to process the information, as well as for the antibiotics to be shipped from the manufacturer. When medical insurances/ prescription insurances cover the antibiotics, there is usually a co-pay. Sometimes this is just to your dental office, which covers the costs to your dentist for the antibiotic to be placed, such as sterilization of the instruments necessary. Sometimes, your insurance requires a separate copay that is either sent to them or to the manufacturer. How much the copay is and how it is split depends upon your particular insurance plan. As patients demand more from their medical insurances, more plans will start to cover these antibiotics.

When your scaling and root planning has been completed, your follow-up appointment is set. This is usually one month later. Your follow-up appointment is to check how well your gums are responding to treatment as well as how you are doing with your home care. Some offices will have different time frames; however, I have found that a month works well for my patients. It is long enough time for healing to have started, but short enough that we can help you improve your home care for any areas that you are missing before bacteria can start to do damage again.

At your follow-up appointment, any areas where you have had plaque and calculus reform are cleaned again. This is much more comfortable than the scaling and root planning because you will have much less debris. Your gums and their healing as well as your level of home care are assessed. This is also the appointment where your teeth are polished. The delay between scaling and root planning and the polishing gives your gums a chance to snug back up to your teeth so that the grit from the polishing paste does not get into your freshly cleaned out pockets.

What should you expect with this? During the actual scaling and root planning, it can be uncomfortable. The stuff being removed, calculus in particular, can be rough and scratchy, kind of like sand. If you have a lot of calculus, your dentist or hygienist may be able to show you one of the larger pieces that is removed for you. You can choose to be numb for the scaling and root planning.

Afterward, expect your gums to be sore and sensitive. They were already inflamed from the infection. Cleaning everything out presses on them and stretches them so the instruments can get into your pockets and the debris removed scratches the inside of the pockets. And now that you do not have plaque and calculus in your pockets, acidic and spicy foods can get down in there and irritate the already inflamed area. The worst of this is usually the first twenty-four to forty-eight hours. Warm salt water rinses can help to sooth your gums as well as wash away acids from foods. Most people do not need any kind of pain medication, however, some will use over the counter treatments. Rarely is the discomfort severe enough to prescription pain medications.

Your teeth may also become sensitive, particularly to cold, hot, and/ or sweet. Tooth sensitivity may appear right away or it may be delayed. In either case, the cause of it is the newly exposed root surface. The root surface of your teeth is much more sensitive to cold, hot, and sweet than your enamel, the surface of the top part of your tooth. This is because the root surface is porous, so hot, cold, and sweet can get through your tooth to the nerve faster. This will usually decrease with time; however desensitizing tooth pastes can aid the process. When your sensitivity happens right away after your scaling and root planning, it is because the debris that was on your teeth was insulating them, kind of like wearing a winter jacket. When sensitivity occurs later, it is due to the inflammation and swelling of your gums subsiding, so the root surface is not being covered by the swollen gums any more.

There are several options to help you if you have sensitivity after scaling and root planning. There are sensitivity reducing tooth pastes which work in several ways depending upon which one you choose. There are both over the counter and prescription sensitivity tooth pastes. Which is right for you is best discussed with your dentist or hygienist. There are over the counter sensitivity strips that can help if you have one or a few teeth that are sensitive. There are also desensitizing rinses. There are also prescription products that your dentist can write a prescription for or may be applied at your dentist's office. There is also the possibility that the calculus and other debris were removed from a cavity, which would be best alleviated by a restoration on the tooth such as a filling or crown.

Any sensitivity should dissipate as your gums continue to heal; however, if you have sensitivity that persists or worsens, it is best to check in with your dentist, whether it be your teeth or your gums. Remember, some sensitivity is normal.

Scaling and root planning is just the first step in treating your periodontal disease. It is a very important step because it removes the bacteria and debris that you cannot remove at home. The thing is, scaling and root planning is not the only step in treating this disease. You will need periodic maintenance cleanings at your dentist's office and you will have to take care of your teeth at home as well.

The periodic maintenance cleanings do need to be more often than the preventative, prophylactic cleanings. After scaling and root planning, the bacteria can build back up to harmful levels. Most of the time, this takes about ninety days. If your home care is on

the lesser end, or you have other medical issues, it may

be faster. If you have exceptional home care it may be

slower. Ninety days is the average, so your timing will

usually start there and then be adjusted to your needs.

All of this professional care, even though it is a

necessary part of controlling your periodontal disease,

is only about thirty percent of the success of treatment.

We clean your teeth four times a year. You need to

clean them every day.

How to take care of your teeth

Home care is the key to success. This is not just for periodontal disease, but for all dental treatment. How well you maintain the cleanliness of your mouth at home determines how long your dental work will last, and how long your teeth will last. That is especially so when it comes to periodontal disease, where seventy percent of the success of treatment is how well you maintain your teeth at home.

Taking care of your teeth now that you have periodontal disease is going to be much more involved than it was before. Remember, what you had been doing is what got you in the position you are in now. So things need to change. If you do not want your periodontal disease to get worse, if you want to keep your teeth, something has to change

You probably already have a manual tooth brush. If anything, you probably were given one at your dentist's office. Even if you are already using an electronic brush or are planning to buy one, the manual brush is still an important tool in your arsenal to combat the bacteria. If anything, it is much easier to carry a manual brush with you than an electronic brush. Carry it in your purse or briefcase; take it in a lunch bag; keep it in your desk or locker, even in your car so that you can clean your teeth for touchups between your main cleanings at home.

The key to a manual brush is how you use it. Most people that have normal dexterity and use of their hands can adequately clean their teeth with a manual tooth brush and floss. Most people do not. That is why a powered brush will help you, and I will review these next.

There are specific techniques for brushing with different techniques being best at different stages of life. This is what I recommend for my periodontally challenged patients such as yourself. This is a start, and, of course, working with your dentist and hygienist is recommended so that they can modify this technique to be most beneficial to you.

Think of your teeth as the world's finest hardwood floors and your gums as the most expensive cabinets in the world. Your mouth is where you eat your food, so you can think of a very fancy kitchen. Now, you want to show off your floors and keep them clean, and you need to get the dust bunnies out from where the cabinets overhang the floors without damaging the cabinets and thoroughly cleaning your floors. So you angle your broom to get under the cabinets and wiggle it gently in short little back and forth strokes to get the dust bunnies out, then nice loinger strokes across the floors.

Now to your teeth. Start with a soft or extra soft tooth brush, remember, you do not want to damage your gums. Firm tooth brushes are not for teeth, they are for grout and cleaning the wheels on your car. You need soft or extra soft. These actually flex into the deeper spaces between your teeth better and are gentler for your gums. You can completely clean with a soft or extra soft tooth brush. It takes a bit longer, at least two minutes, probably more while you are learning how to clean everywhere. The key is thorough but gentle.

Angle the brush under your gums, just as you would angle a broom to reach under the cabinets, about 45 degrees. Using short, gentle, strokes, wiggle back and forth under the gums, then, using longer strokes, sweep from your gums to the biting surface of your teeth. I know this is different from the usual little circles or back and forth that is would normally be recommended, but if that was working for you, you would not have developed periodontal disease.

A helpful tool when you are first learning this technique is a disclosing agent. Disclosing agents dye your plaque a bright color so that it is easier for you to see to remove it. These come in several colors, red is the most common. There are two common forms, liquid and tablets. For home use, I recommend the tablets, mostly because the liquid can be messy and both of these can stain, so the less messy option is usually better. Disclosing tablets are available over the counter, but some pharmacies keep them behind the counter or have to order them for you. To use the tablets, take one, chew it up and swish with water for a minute, then expectorate (spit it out). Please note, you will want to do this in an easily cleaned area, especially when first using it.

I usually recommend starting out using the disclosing tablet first, before brushing and flossing. Then keep cleaning your teeth until you have removed all of the brightly colored plaque. Then, once you have mastered that, try cleaning your teeth first, then use the disclosing tablet to see what you have missed and concentrate on those areas. Many people find that they tend to miss the same areas that they have the deepest infected pockets.

While a manual brush and floss can remove all of the food and plaque on your teeth, a mechanical brush can make it much easier for you. This is especially true for people that have limited use of their hands, such as from arthritis, of if you ever have to brush someone else's teeth for them.

Mechanical brushes do a lot of the work for you. In most cases, you just have to move the brush along your teeth and just make sure all areas are cleaned. It does the actual brushing.

There are three that I recommend for my patients, and I base my recommendation on each patient's needs. Your dentist and hygienist can help you to select which is best for you.

The three I currently recommend for my patients are the Oral-B professional series, the Sonicare diamond clean, and the Rotadent. There are positives and negatives for each, which is why I make my recommendations based upon your needs.

The Oral-B has the greatest selection of brush heads for different purposes. It is also a fairly powerful brush. It has a little red light in it that lights up if you start to brush too hard; I personally feel that his is its best feature. There are video tutorials on their website to show you how to use it, so the quick overview is to gently guide the brush along your teeth at the gum line and across the biting surfaces, allowing it to do the work. The built in timer will direct you when to change areas. As a side note, it has been my finding that the orthodontic brush head stands up to brackets better for my patients that are going through orthodontics better than other brands of brushes.

The Sonicare diamond clean has gentler vibrations that can be easier for people who do not like as much vibration, but it is also a bit more work for you. Sonicare has excellent usage tutorial videos on their website. The summary is that you hold the brush against you teeth for a few seconds, and then move to the next area with a little overlap. So your motion is more start and stop. Remember to allow the brush to do that actual work.

The Rotadent is the gentlest of the three from a vibration standpoint. It uses a motion similar to the polisher used at dental offices. The Rotadent also has the finest bristles of the three, so they can reach further between your teeth and under your gums. The Rotadent has excellent tutorial videos on their website for use instructions. The usage summary is that you slowly move the brush over all surfaces of your teeth. Because the brush head is smaller than either of the others, you will have to move more to clean every surface.

All of these work very well for different people, which is why I recommend discussing them with your dentist or hygienist to see which will work best for you. These are the three that I recommend most often, there are other mechanical brushes out there which your dentist may recommend if that is what will work best for you.

After you have brushed, cleaning between your teeth is the next step. So no, you do not need to floss, but you do still need to clean between your teeth. Exactly which way will work best for you is best discussed with your dentist or hygienist, but these are the basics.

Floss has gotten a bad rap recently. Someone in the news media decided to announce that there are no studies that show that floss itself can prevent periodontal disease or cavities. While this is true, there is a huge however attached. There are no studies specifically showing that floss alone can prevent cavities and periodontal disease, HOWEVER, there are numerous studies that show plaque removal does prevent periodontal disease and that floss does remove plaque between teeth where brushes cannot reach. There are no studies for floss alone because it needs brushing to completely clean your teeth and brushing needs a way to clean between your teeth, so it is not either one alone. That is why there are no solo studies for floss.

So, how do you floss? Many people just snap the floss in and out of the space between teeth, in and out, once and done. That only cleans a single stripe on the side of your tooth that is about the width of a pencil line, and it also runs the risk of snapping the floss into your gums and cutting them.

To floss properly, and clean the maximum surface area, take your length of floss (about 12-18 inches) and wrap the ends around your fingers, more on one hand than the other. Using a sawing motion, pass the floss through the point where your teeth touch. Then pull the floss against the side of one tooth and slide up and down below your gums and up to where your teeth touch. Slide several times, and then repeat on the tooth next to it before coming back up through where your teeth touch and moving to the next contact. When you move to the next area, unwind some floss from one hand and onto the other so you have a fresh area of floss to clean with. This is why I recommend winding more onto one hand at the beginning, so that you move through the floss to clean each area. Just as it takes time to learn to brush differently; it will take longer than you are used to at first. I recommend doing this in front of a mirror until you are comfortable and able to easily maneuver through all areas of your mouth.

Floss holders are devices that allow you to use your own floss, which you change out between uses. Because you put the floss on, you get to pick the type of floss and you set the tension on the floss. These are good if you have limited dexterity or if you need to floss someone else's teeth. By setting the tension of the floss yourself, you can make sure it is not too tight to pull against the side of your tooth.

Floss picks are pre-threaded floss holders so you do not select your own floss and you do not set the tension on the floss. They are usually fairly tightly set, so it is difficult to curve the floss against your tooth. These are great for carrying around with you, but not as good as a floss holder where you put the floss on yourself.

Interproximal brushes are another aid for cleaning between your teeth. These are particularly useful for people that have some space there, such as a complete gap between your teeth or even just space between where your teeth touch and your gums. When you have spaces, it can be more difficult to clean your teeth with floss as larger pieces of food can become stuck in the space and floss might not be able to pull it out.

There are two main manual types of interproximal brushes. End tuft brushes have one or a few tufts of bristles at the end but otherwise look like a regular tooth brush. There are also interproximal brushes that look like a segment of pipe cleaner on a handle. There are also interproximal brush tips for some of the mechanical brushes. All are used similarly. Gently push the bristles through between your teeth and wiggle. If you have a mechanical brush, remember to let the brush do the work for you.

Another way to clean between your teeth is with water irrigation systems. Water irrigation systems use a stream of water to wash out the areas between your teeth.

There are two main types of irrigation systems, interrupted pulse and continuous flow. The interrupted pulse, most prominent being the Sonicare Water Floss, use one to three quick bursts of water to push debris and plaque out from between your teeth. Continuous flow irrigators have an uninterrupted stream of water that washes out debris and plaque between your teeth and around the gum line. The most prominent continuous stream system is Waterpik; however, several companies make these.

There is a learning curve with water irrigation, mostly learning how to clean everywhere without soaking your bathroom. Both Sonicare and Waterpik have excellent tutorial videos on their websites for using their devices.

I do want to make note that Waterpik has a tip specifically designed for use in periodontal disease areas. This tip has a soft rubber point that is made to slide between your teeth and gums to reach further into the deep periodontally infected pockets. I know that Waterpik has it noted in their directions, but it is worth noting again here, even though their regular above the gums tip is most effective at higher settings (above a 6 on their machines), the periodontal, under the gums tip must be kept at the lowest setting or you run the risk of damaging yourself. So if you use this tip, keep the machine on the lightest setting.

A note for people who smoke and those that drink alcohol. These two things contribute to periodontal disease. Smoking, besides being carcinogenic, has other complicating factors specific for periodontal disease. Nicotine is a vasoconstrictor. This means that it causes your blood vessels to become smaller. This limits your body's ability to heal after periodontal procedures. It also disguises your periodontal disease, because the disease has to be much worse for a smoker's gums to actively bleed when brushing or flossing. The periodontal infection is still there, but it does not bleed as much due to the vasoconstriction. Alcohol is an irritant to gum tissue. This irritation can make healing take longer as well. It also can dry the tissues out, again making healing take longer. If you can, stop these behaviors. If you cannot stop completely, try to cut down, or at least stop while you are in healing phases of treatment. Your gums will thank you.

Your dentist and hygienist will help you to discover what will work best for you. This is just an overview of the many options available. The key is finding what works best for your teeth and your gums.

Cleaning and taking care of your teeth when you have periodontal disease is going to take longer than you are used to, especially while you are learning new techniques. Know that, with time, and practice, you will become faster; just make sure that you remain gentle but thorough. Remember, you only need to clean the teeth you want to keep and seventy percent of the success of treatment depends upon you.

The Oral –Systemic Connection

So now you know a bit about what periodontal disease is, how it is treated, and how to maintain your teeth at home. This section is why periodontal disease is so important.

There is no cure for periodontal disease, only prevention or control. The closest current option to a cure is to remove all of your teeth. For some people, especially severe cases, that might be the best option. For most people who have periodontal disease, control to maintain it at its current level is the better option.

I am telling you this because periodontal disease damages more than just your mouth, it does damage throughout your body. Even removal of your teeth can not undo the damage that has been caused elsewhere.

Periodontal disease is an inflammatory disease. Yes, it starts with an infection. The start, when it was gingivitis, was just infection, but it is the inflammation that does the real damage.

The inflammation from periodontal disease is what causes your bone and gums to detach from your teeth, but the thing is the inflammation does not stay just in your mouth. The inflammation spreads throughout your body while also causing damage to your gums that allows periodontal disease bacteria into your blood stream, so they spread and cause even more damage elsewhere.

The big one, the one that affects everyone that has periodontal disease is that you are now at increased risk of heart attacks, strokes, arteriosclerosis, and other cardiovascular diseases. These are all part of the same problem, just different areas of the body: inflammation of and plaque in your blood stream. Do you know why they call the buildup inside blood vessels plaque? I will give you a great big hint: it has the same bacteria in it as the plaque on your teeth.

Your increased risk of cardiovascular diseases is directly linked to the severity of your periodontal disease. Early periodontal disease has a slightly higher risk. Severe periodontal disease has a greatly increased risk. There is such a high correlation between severe periodontal disease and cardiovascular disease that I recommend all of my severely infected patients to seek evaluation by their physicians or a cardiologist. A recent study, the Bale-Doneen study, has shown not just a correlation between periodontal disease and cardiovascular disease but a direct causation. Periodontal disease is one of the causes of cardiovascular disease.

If that is not scary enough, let us look at some of the other diseases that periodontal disease plays a role in.

Diabetes is a complex group of diseases that all result in the same end, elevated levels of glucose in your blood. There are three main types of diabetes: type I, type II, and gestational, with more types being studied and defined. They have different causes. Type I is caused by an autoimmune disease that destroys the cells in the pancreas that make insulin, a hormone that regulates your body's use of sugars. Type II and gestational are the result of the body not being able to respond to the insulin hormone. All of them cause sugar to buildup in your blood. This sugar sticks to your red blood cells which makes the red blood cells rough and scratchy, which scratches the inside of your blood vessels and causes inflammation and damage throughout your body.

Now take periodontal disease, an infection that causes inflammation and add that to it. It makes a spiral downward. First, periodontal disease, and chronic inflammation from it, is a risk factor for developing type II diabetes. For all types of diabetes, uncontrolled periodontal disease makes your diabetes harder to control. Uncontrolled diabetes makes your periodontal disease harder to treat and control. They work together against you.

Pre-term and low birthweight babies would seem to be something that just the child's mother would need to worry about, but it is really a matter for both parents. Pre-term and low birthweights predispose the child to numerous health problems, even later in life, so the care of these children can be much more complicated and expensive. Expectant

mothers that have periodontal disease are at greater

risk of having pre-term and low birthweight babies.

Think about it, it is hard enough for your body to grow

another human being. Now, try doing it while fighting a

chronic infection. Add on that the hormones of

pregnancy make it easier for you to develop gingivitis,

the start of periodontal disease. Dads, you are not off

the hook on this; the bacteria that cause periodontal

disease are contagious.

It may seem that I am picking on issues that

affect women, but osteoporosis can happen to anyone.

It is just more common in women. I will first tell you a

bit about osteoporosis. It causes your bones to become

brittle. You have two sets of cells that work on your

bone. One set puts down new bone, the other takes old

bone away. In osteoporosis, the cells that take bone

away are going faster than the cells that put down new bone. So overall, you wind up losing bone slowly from everywhere. Periodontal disease causes bone loss in and of itself. When you have both, they go even faster. That is bad enough itself, but the medications used to control osteoporosis cause increased complication rates for periodontal disease treatments. So you have two diseases that make each other progress faster and the treatment for one disease makes treatment of the other more risky.

Alzheimer's disease is a horrible disease. I know. I have seen it. I have watched my patients that have it deteriorate. I have watched their loved ones do their best to care for someone slowly slipping away from them. My fiancé's mother has it. Yes, I know this disease. While periodontal disease does not cause

Alzheimer's disease directly, its chronic inflammation is a risk factor for it and can make it progress faster.

Have I scarred you yet? Well, let's make it even worse.

Cancer. The "Big C." Periodontal disease increases your risk of getting cancer. New research is showing that, while periodontal disease is not likely to be the cause of cancer itself, the inflammation from it allows other carcinogens (cancer causing chemicals) to get deeper into your tissues easier.

This is why your dentist and hygienist are so concerned about periodontal disease. Yes, of course, we care about your teeth. But this, this is why periodontal disease gets the "silent killer" label. It creeps up on you and causes so many other problems that you would not connect to it, unless you are told about the connection.

That is where you can do great things to help your own health. Getting periodontal disease under control can help you in a multitude of ways and reduce your risk of multiple other diseases.

Adjunctive and Advanced procedures

Adjunctive and advanced procedures go beyond the basic minimal treatment. There are several purposes for these. Some, such as antibiotics, help you heal faster with better results. Some, such as surgery, are for areas that are not responding to regular treatment or sometimes reverse the damage than has been done.

Directly placed antibiotics are antibiotics that are put directly into your infected periodontal pockets. These antibiotics are often placed in conjunction with either your scaling and root planning or other procedures. These help your gums to heal faster and better than they would without the antibiotics. First, antibiotics kill bacteria. Bacteria are what start the whole periodontal disease process. Second, the directly placed antibiotics fill space. They block food and debris from getting into your freshly cleaned pockets. Third, they can modify the way your body responds to what bacteria are present so that your body's attack does less harm to itself and decreases your gums and bone detaching from your teeth. So, not only do the antibiotics kill bacteria, but they also physically block bacteria and plaque from getting back into the deep areas and decrease the inflammation that the bacteria cause.

There are three main brands of directly placed antibiotics: Periochip, Arestin, and Atridox. Periochip was the first, and while it still exists, is not used very often anymore because the others can be more effective. Arestin and Atridox are similar in that they are both in the same family of antibiotics, the tetracycline family. The techniques for placement of these two antibiotics are different. Arestin is a powder when it is placed that turns into a gel then a firm wax like solid. Atridox starts as a gel that turns into a firm wax-like solid. Both slowly dissolve over about two weeks with antibacterial activity for about four weeks.

I have used both Arestin and Atridox in my practice and they each have their benefits. I have found similar responses to both. Atridox, by the manner in which it is placed, allows for flowing between areas, whereas Arestin is placed individually site by site. For some patients, Atridox can be more cost effective because we can flow the material into some borderline sites adjacent to areas that are definitively infected. For some patients, their medical insurance may cover Arestin, dependent upon what their medical prescription plan's coverages are.

In the case of any of the directly placed antibiotics, it is important to follow home care directions closely. The main thing is to not dislodge the antibiotic. Your dentist or hygienist will discuss home care with you. Usually the home care includes not using a mechanical tooth brush, not using a water irrigation system, and not flossing or using a tooth pick in the treated area for a certain amount of time following the placement of the antibiotic. You still brush manually and still normally clean teeth in non-treatment areas.

The directly placed antibiotics are adjunctive treatments, they help you heal faster with better results, but they cannot treat your periodontal disease alone. For this reason, most dental insurances do not cover directly placed antibiotics; however, because these are antibiotics for an infection, some medical prescription insurances will cover these directly placed antibiotics; covering the antibiotic itself. The antibiotic will still need to be placed in the office. There is usually some kind of co-pay. As more patients demand coverage by their medical insurance, coverage will improve.

Perio-endoscopic procedures are non-surgical treatments for periodontal disease that use a special magnification system called and endoscope to magnify and show the deep areas of your infected pockets on a computer screen. This device allows your dentist or hygienist to see the roots of your teeth above the bone without having to cut your gums to move the gums out of the way. This enhanced visibility allows any complicated areas of your roots to be seen so that they can be treated better.

The most common use of the perio-endoscope is in areas that are not responding well to initial treatments. Sometimes it is used alone for diagnostic purposes. Sometimes it is used in conjunction with other treatments, such as ensuring all debris, plaque, and calculus are removed from areas that have more complex anatomy. This is a way to try to not do surgery unless you absolutely need it.

Laser assisted procedures use a laser for several purposes. First, the laser can be used to help disinfect your periodontal pockets. This, just like the directly placed antibiotics, helps you heal better and faster. Second, there are laser procedures that can help you re-grow your lost tissue attachment. Called laser Assisted New attachment Procedures, LANAP for short, stimulate your bone and gums to re-grow in areas that have been lost. So far, everything that I have covered has been to stop your periodontal disease from getting worse, this is one of the treatments designed to reverse it. The thing is, LANAP does not work on everyone. A lot of it depends upon you. Your periodontal disease needs to be stabilized and you need to be able to keep your mouth meticulously clean for this to work. On top of that, it took you a while to lose your bone and gums; it can take a while to see results from LANAP to get them back.

And now we will delve into the periodontal surgeries. These are surgery and are more advanced procedures. I do some of these surgeries in my office myself, others I refer to a specialist, either a periodontist or an oral surgeon.

Periodontists are dentists that have had additional training to specify their skills to just the treatment of periodontal disease and the results of it, such as tooth loss. I usually will send a patient to a periodontist if their infection is not responding to treatment, if a patient is ready for some advanced treatments such as grafting, or if a patient has very severe periodontal disease and wants to do everything that they can to maintain their teeth as long as possible. Oral surgeons are dentists who have received specialized training in surgical procedures of your face and jaw. I usually refer to an oral surgeon for bone and gum grafting and implant placements as well as extractions. These two specialists are there to help you when your care needs to be more complex.

Gingivectomy is a surgical procedure that removes excessive gum tissue. This is usually for when your gums are swollen to an extent that you cannot clean your teeth well. It gets the excess, swollen tissue out of the way. It can also be used to cosmetically re-shape your gums, such as if your gums are uneven one side to another when you smile.

Clinical crown lengthening is a surgical procedure that permanently removes some of the surrounding and supporting bone and gum tissue around a tooth when the tooth has a different problem, like a cavity or a crack, that goes below your gum line. In these circumstances, it is necessary to move the gums and bone out of the way so that the tooth can be fixed. When a tooth has an issue like this, that goes under the gums, the alternative to reshaping your gums and bone is to remove the tooth. The gum and bone that is blocking access to the area is removed and a smooth transition is made away from that area, which may include adjacent teeth. This smooth transition makes it easier for you to keep the area clean after it has healed.

When you have very deep periodontal pockets and you have had bone loss, then you have the option of an apically positioned flap. In this surgery, your gums are cut and pulled away from your teeth and bone, then re-attached at a lower position, further down the root of the tooth. This procedure preserves your gum tissue, but just moves it so that you no longer have very deep, hard to clean areas. The whole purpose of this is to make it easier for you to keep your teeth clean and have access to all areas of your teeth.

Surgical scaling is a surgery to clean difficult to access areas, areas that are difficult for your dentist and hygienist to reach even with their specialized instruments. In surgical scaling, your gums are cut and moved away from your teeth and bone. The teeth are then thoroughly cleaned, even the difficult areas, and your dentist or periodontist can directly see that everything has been cleaned off of your teeth. Your gums are then put back where they were and held in place by stitches until they heal. Sometimes this is combined with apically positioned flaps, sometimes it is combined with grafting.

Grafts are a way for you to regain tissues that you have lost. Gum tissue grafts give you back lost gum tissue. Bone grafts give you back lost bone. There are two sources for gingival grafts: somewhere else in your mouth or donated tissue. Both work and which is best for you would best be discussed with your dentist, surgeon, or periodontist. Bone grafts have several sources. Your bone tends to work best, but requires another area to have your bone harvested from. There is donated bone, there are animal bone sources and there are completely artificially made bone matrix substitutes. Each works best under certain circumstances and what will work best for you will be discussed with your dentist, surgeon, or periodontist.

The intention of all of the grafts is to put back what you have lost.

For all adjunctive and advanced treatment options, how well you take care of your teeth greatly determines your outcomes. Remember, 70% of the success of treatment is from your home care. In the case of these options, it is even more critical. The best candidates for advanced procedures, especially those designed to re-gain attachment to your teeth, have 15 % or fewer sites that have active inflammation.

Dentistry is an ever evolving science, and new techniques and materials are coming out every day. These presented here are just the beginning of what is possible for your treatment and are the most common of the adjunctive and advanced procedures. Which options will work best for you and your mouth is best discussed with your dentist and hygienist. Every mouth

is unique and so is every treatment plan.

Peri-implantitis

Peri-implantitis is the same disease as periodontal disease; it is just around a dental implant instead of a tooth. Dental implants are a tooth replacement that is currently the closest to having your natural teeth back. From your standpoint, you treat your dental implants just like teeth.

For your reference, I have already written a guide book about dental implants for you. The Patient's Guide to Dental Implants is available on Amazon.

Just like teeth, you can get infection in the pocket around your implant. Because the implant is attached to you a little differently than a tooth is, the progress of peri-implantitis may be slower than it is around your natural teeth, however, it is more complicated to treat.

Peri-implantitis is diagnosed just as periodontal disease is, with a combination of measurements, radiographs, and visual examination. It may also use a resonance frequency device that measures how stable your implant is in your bone.

The difficulty in treating peri-implantitis is due to the shape and texture of the implant. The surface of your implant that was in your bone is rough. It is supposed to be rough. The roughness encourages your bone to fuse to the implant and gives your bone more to hold onto. On top of this, most implants have a threaded or other convoluted shape that holds it in place when it is initially healing. These are great when we want your implant to heal into your bone. The difficulty is only if you lose that bony attachment and these rough, complex shapes become exposed in the pocket so bacteria can stick to it. It is almost impossible to clean the implant surface without a perio-endoscope or surgery to move the gums out of the way.

The full process of treatment for peri-implantitis can be very involved, depending upon the severity of the infection and amount of bone and gum loss. It will usually start with a regular, non-surgical scaling. The purpose of this is to reduce inflammation for better visibility and results of subsequent treatment. After several weeks, you would have a surgical scaling where your gums are cut away from your implant so all areas can be accessed. With your gums out of the way, your implant is able to be scaled across areas above your bone. Then the implant surface is disinfected and cleaned chemically to remove any microscopic areas of bacteria. Sometimes bone grafting is done at this time to help replace bone that you have lost. Then your gums are stitched closed and allowed to heal.

Once the surgery has been completed, how well you keep the area clean is the largest factor in your results. Remember, you paid for that implant; you need to maintain it to keep it. Just as periodontal disease can result in the loss of teeth, peri-implantitis can result in the loss of your implant.

Conclusion

Periodontal disease is the big bad guy of dentistry. It is the silent killer, in more ways than one, and you do not feel it until it is in the later stages.

It is bad. I cannot stress that enough. And neither can your dentist and hygienist.

Having periodontal disease throughout your mouth is the same as having an infected open wound the size of your palm. If you had that on your leg, you would treat it. But this is tucked in around your teeth and spread out. You don't see it. You can only see the symptoms of it, and many of those are subtle. Your dentist and hygienist see it. They know how devastating it is for patients. They know how sad it is for a patient to have a tooth just fall out. They know the financial strain of an insurance refusing to pay for a crown because the tooth is periodontally compromised. They now what it is like to see a patient's health deteriorate with the systemic complications that are related to periodontal disease.

And there is hope. Periodontal disease can be controlled. Your dentist and hygienist can help. Further bone loss and gum loss can be prevented. Controlling your periodontal disease reduces your risks for systemic diseases.

Your dentist and hygienist can help you get your periodontal disease under control. They can remove the calculus and bacteria that you cannot and give you a fresh start to maintain what you have. They get your teeth clean and you maintain them that way.

My hope for you is that you will take this information to get the care that you need. Periodontal disease is a destructive, chronic, inflammatory disease, but it can be controlled. It will take some work on your part as well as your dental team's help. It can be done.

I would love to see every one you in my office, but I also know that Apopka, Florida may be a bit out of your way. There are many excellent dentists throughout the U.S. and around the world. I recommend that you start your periodontal treatment with your regular dentist that you are comfortable with. Discuss your options. If you need additional resources, I recommend your local dental society, the American Dental Association, and the American Academy of Periodontology. While there are many great dentists that are part of these organizations, there are also many great dentists who are not, which is why I recommend starting locally and finding a dentist that you are comfortable with.

I wish you happy and healthy smiles for a lifetime.

Dental Dictionary

Acute Necrotizing Ulcerative Gingivitis – a severe type of infection of the gum tissue that causes the gingiva to die and ulcerate. This is typically very painful and bleeds spontaneously. This is abbreviated as ANUG and is also called trench mouth.

Advanced and adjunctive procedures – these are procedures that are secondary to the first line of treatment. This includes placement of antibiotics directly into the area, use of perio-endocscopes, laser based procedures, and surgical procedures. These procedures may be done in your regular dentist's office or may be at a specialist's office.

Alzheimer's disease – a degenerative neurological disease that causes loss of memory with patients progressively losing more and more of their memory and other abilities.

Anesthetic gel – a numbing agent applied to the surface of your gums. This typically numbs just the first couple millimeters of your gum tissue. Spray on versions also exist.

Arteriosclerosis – hardening of your arteries, often caused by cholesterol and plaque, a type of cardiovascular disease.

Biofilm – the combination of bacteria, bacterial secretions, and food particles that enhances the bacteria's bond to the tooth surface.

Bisphosphonate medications – medicines used to treat both osteoporosis and some cancers. This is a form of chemotherapy. These medications have been linked to increased risk of complications after certain dental treatments, including the treatment of periodontal disease.

Calculus – calcified plaque. Due to calcification, this cannot be removed with tooth brush and floss, requiring specialized instruments to remove.

Carcinogen – a chemical known to cause cancer.

Cardiovascular disease – disease of the heart and vascular system.

Deep cleaning – cleanings of your teeth that are more involved than the traditional, preventative, prophylactic cleaning. These can be full mouth debridement, scaling for gingivitis, or scaling and root planing. These deeper types of cleanings are less invasive than the surgical cleanings.

Dental hygienist – a licensed dental professional who's training and care is geared to the cleaning of teeth.

Dental insurance – a product that you purchase or your employer has purchased for you that helps to pay for some dental procedures. Most dental insurances have a cap of how much they will pay in a year and you will usually have a copay, or portion to pay for most procedures.

Dentist – a doctor that has specialized their care to your mouth and other oral structures.

Diabetes – a set of diseases that cause elevated levels of glucose in your blood. Type 1 is an autoimmune disease that causes an organ called the pancreas to stop producing insulin, a hormone that controls the glucose level. Type 2 and gestational diabetes are results of your body not being able to respond to insulin.

Directly placed antibiotics – antibiotics that are placed directly into infected periodontal pockets.

Disclosing agents – a dye that stains plaque and calculus to make it easier for you to see and remove.

Floss – an instrument to clean the interproximal surfaces of teeth.

Furcation – the point where the roots of a tooth meet in a multi-rooted tooth.

General Dentist – your regular dentist that has not specifically limited their practice to one specific area of dentistry.

Gingivitis – inflammation and infection of the gum tissue prior to the onset of periodontal disease. This is a completely reversible condition. No tooth attachment has been lost.

Heart Attack – when your heart stops beating, causing death if the heart cannot be started again.

Infection – an illness that is caused by either bacteria or virus. In the case of periodontal disease, the infection is caused by bacteria.

Inflammation – your body's response to injury and infection. This is a combined effect of immune system as well as healing cells infiltrating the area. Often causes redness, tenderness, and warmth of the area. It is also the mechanism your body uses to wall off infections that it cannot fight. In the case of periodontal disease, this inflammation causes the detachment of your gums and bone from your teeth in an effort to isolate the infection and prevent it spreading.

Interproximal – the surfaces of teeth that are between teeth.

Low birth weight – a baby that is carried to full term, however, it is small for its age. This has been linked to many potential future health issues for the child.

Oral and maxillofacial surgeon – a dentist that has received additional training to specialize their treatment to surgical procedures of the mouth and face.

Osteoporosis – a degenerative condition of the bone where the bone becomes brittle and weak. This is often treated with bisphosphonate medications, which have been linked to complications from dental treatment.

Peri-implantitis – a compound illness that starts as an infection between your dental implant and gums that, combined with your body's inflammation causes implant attachment loss to the gingiva and bone as well as systemic complications. This is the same infection that causes periodontal disease around teeth.

Periodontal charting – measurements of the attachment level of gingiva to a tooth and condition of the gum tissue.

Periodontal disease – a compound illness that starts as an infection between your teeth and gums that, combined with your body's inflammation, causes tooth attachment loss to gingiva and bone as well as systemic complications. Also known as periodontitis. This same infection is also causative of peri-implantitis around dental implants.

Periodontal ligament – a fibrous attachment between your jaw bone and gums and teeth. This acts as both a shock absorber and as a mechanism for proprioception.

Periodontal maintenance cleanings – periodic cleanings that maintain the health of your mouth and help to prevent the accumulation of bacteria to levels where they can become detrimental.

Periodontist – a dentist that has received additional training to specialize their practice to just the treatment of periodontal disease.

Perio-probe – an instrument used to measure the depth of a periodontal pocket as well as other measurements in the mouth.

Plaque – a biofilm of bacteria, food particles, and bacterial secretions that sticks to the surface of your teeth. In larger quantities, this causes gingivitis and periodontal disease. The combination of bacteria, food particles, and bacterial secretions causes it to be sticky such that it will not rinse off and needs to be physically removed. This can be removed by brushing and flossing.

Pocket – the space between your gums and your tooth above the attachment of the gums to the tooth on an infected area.

Pre-term babies – babies that are not carried to the full term of pregnancy, also called premature or preemies. This has been linked to a multitude of potential health issues for the child.

Prophylactic cleaning – this is a preventative cleaning. It is for patients that have healthy mouths to prevent the onset of dental and gingival diseases such as carries, gingivitis, and periodontal disease.

Proprioception – your body's ability to locate parts of itself in space, how you know where your hand is such that you can touch your nose with your eyes closed.

Radiographs – commonly called x-rays, these are imaged used to evaluate the health of your teeth and bone.

Tooth root – the portion of the tooth that is meant to anchor your tooth into your bone.

Scaling and root planing – a cleaning in the deep cleaning category, this is the most common front line treatment for periodontal disease. This involves cleaning the root surfaces of debris, plaque and calculus deep under the gum line, beyond where your home cleaning can reach. The goal of this is to reduce the bacteria to a level that no longer causes progression of periodontal disease. Scaling is the removal of debris from the tooth, root planing is smoothing the surface of the tooth to make it easier to clean and more difficult for bacteria to adhere to the tooth surface.

Scaling for gingivitis – cleaning in the deep cleaning category, this cleaning is for patients that have gingivitis generalized throughout their mouth and more debris, plaque, and calculus than can be removed with a prophylactic cleaning.

Sulcus – the space between your gums and your tooth above the attachment of the gums to the tooth in a non-infected area.

Tooth attachment – your body's mechanism of holding in your teeth, called the periodontal ligament.

Ulcer – an open wound that is difficult to heal.

Ultrasonic cleaner – a mechanical device for cleaning teeth that uses sound waves above human hearing to break up debris, plaque, and calculus so that it can be rinsed away. The two main types are the Cavitron and Piezo systems.

Vascular system – the arteries and veins that carry blood throughout your heart.

Vasoconstrictor – a chemical that causes your arteries and veins to constrict, which increases your blood pressure and makes your heart work harder.

Water irrigator – a machine that creates a focused stream of water used to augment cleaning your mouth, often intended for cleaning between teeth.

X-rays – a common term used for radiographs, ,x-rays are actually light rays beyond human vision that are used to take radiographs

Acknowledgements

Special thanks to Dr. Ronald J. Trevisani for providing my patients with bone grafts and gingival grafts as well as dental implants and Dr. Thomas Yoon for taking care of my more difficult to treat periodontal disease patients.

Thank you to Dr. Samuel Low, for teaching how treatment of periodontal disease really works in practice.

Last, but not least, a huge thank you to my family, for supporting me through all of my training and being my example patients for so many things.

About the author

Dr. Katrina M. Schroeder is a general dentist in Apopka, Florida. She has been in practice since 2006, seeing patients of all ages and with mouths in all conditions. Dr. Schroeder provides care for all aspects of dentistry, including fillings, cosmetic dentistry, veneers, whitening, crowns, dental implants, and, of course, periodontal disease.

She has studied periodontal disease extensively and strives to make sure that all patients that would benefit from treatment are aware of the options available to them. Periodontal disease is very prevalent and treatment of this infectious, contagious disease is so very important. Dr. Schroeder is dedicated to making sure that her patients know their options for their care and what benefits and detriments of each option are, so that they can make the best decisions for their own health and happiness.

Dr. Schroeder completed her Doctor of Dental Medicine (D.M.D.) at the University of Florida College of Dentistry and her Bachelors of Science at the University of Central Florida in Biology with a Chemistry minor and University Honors.

When not with her patients, Dr. Schroeder enjoys spending time with her family, reading (usually about dentistry) and biking. She participates in several charity running events each year. Her hobbies include writing, painting, and restoring antique and classic cars.

$20 Examination and Consultation

This is an offer for anyone who has read through this book. For those of you in the Central Florida area, I am offering you a consultation and examination to review your treatment options at my office for just $20. (Dental codes D0150 and D0274)

Please bring your copy of this book with you to your appointment to redeem this offer. Offer is good through December 31, 2021. You may share your book with multiple people; just have them bring it in with them for their initial consultations too.

Schroeder Dental Group

200 North park Avenue

Suite A

Apopka FL, 32703

(407) 886-1611

Periodontal disease discussion guide

On my website, www.ThePatientsGuidetoDentistry.com, you can request a discussion guide to take with you to your consultations.

www.ingramcontent.com/pod-product-compliance
Lightning Source LLC
Chambersburg PA
CBHW072103280526
45788CB00006B/2378